CHENNAI MINDS
THERAPY WITHOUT THERAPIST SERIES

COGNITIVE BEHAVIOUR THERAPY FOR DEPRESSION

<u>Dr. Radhika MRCPsych MSc (Psych) CCT(UK)</u>
Consultant Psychiatrist
CHENNAI MINDS
<u>www.chennaiminds.com</u>
<u>drradhika@chennaiminds.com</u>

TABLE OF CONTENTS

INTRODUCTION
COGNITIVE BEHAVIOUR THERAPY (CBT)
NEGATIVE AUTOMATIC THOUGHTS (SAD THOUGHTS)
IDENTIFY YOUR SAD THOUGHTS
MANAGE YOUR SAD THOUGHTS
IDENTIFY AND CHALLENGE YOUR THINKING ERRORS
SELF HELP EXERCISES
- Dedicated worry times
- Imagery
- Name the thought/ name the feeling
- Mindfulness
- Breathe mindfully
- Progressive muscle relaxation
- Pleasant activities
- Grounding 5

EXPAND YOUR SOCIAL CONNECTIONS
MANAGE YOUR EXPECTATIONS
IDENTIFY YOUR COMMUNICATION STYLE
COMMUNICATE EFFECTIVELY
CONCLUSION
FLASHCARDS FOR POSITIVE AFFIRMATIONS

DISCLAIMER

THIS BOOK IS PART OF A SERIES OF THERAPY BOOKS AIMED TOWARDS SELF HELP FOR DEPRESSION AND OTHER MENTAL ILLNESSES. THIS SERIES IS NOT A SUBSTITUTE FOR PROFESSIONAL PSYCHIATRIC HELP.

No part of this book should be reproduced, copied or distributed. Copyright lies with CHENNAI MINDS

FOREWORD

Self-help is difficult to define but there are no doubts that this is a popular way of seeking help, especially when one is reluctant to access specialist help. A sad mood is a common enough experience – no one escapes it. Many times, one is "not in the right mood" "Not interested in doing anything" "feels worthless" and countless such negative mood states. Often, one knows not what to do – that is when one reaches out for Self-help books!

I am a psychiatrist with over three decades of psychiatry practice in a busy clinical service run by a premier NGO in Chennai, the Schizophrenia Research Foundation (SCARF India). Depression is the commonest condition that one sees in practice. Yet, this is the tip of the iceberg – there are tens of thousands of people – of all ages out there – who do not want to see a mental health professional! The stigma rules strong!

Dr. Radhika sets out to reach all those persons who need help but won't access help! When Dr. Radhika returned to India from the UK and started 'Chennai Minds', she felt the strong urge to put out something simple to guide and encourage people to make the change. In this book, which is part of the *Chennai Minds Therapy without Therapists Series*, she attempts to reach hardworking people who want to make the change through their own efforts.

With evidence suggesting that Cognitive Behaviour Therapy is a strong strategy to help with one's depression, this book focuses on all those negative thoughts that bother you! The self-help approach fits well with Cognitive Behaviour Therapy, in which you are encouraged to carry out.

Writing this book for persons with Depression, Dr Radhika says, "it is intended to be a practical guide to understand the how one can help oneself to address the challenges faced by people whose *negative thoughts* that can make the day painful". The aim of this book is to provide in simple language an orientation to the various ways by which you can you identify errors in thinking and neatly illustrates the potential error sources. She encourages you through various means to change the ways you think. She uses very simple language with no technical jargon, enabling several reads through the day. The reader of this book will be able to relate to a lot of what is written, either in oneself or in someone close. I am sure that reading this book will allow you to understand your low moods and encourages you to practice of what could be the beginning of a change process in you.

My congratulations to the author, Dr Radhika, Consultant Psychiatrist, CHENNAI MINDS, at www.chennaiminds.com with best wishes for the onward journey.

Dr R Padmavati
Director
Schizophrenia Research Foundation, (SCARF, India)

ACKNOWLEDGEMENTS

My heartfelt gratitude to my best friend. You stood by me, encouraged me, believed in my strengths, rekindled my passion for writing, guided me and supported me through and through in writing this therapy series.

Words cannot express my gratitude and so this book series is dedicated to you, my friend.

I thank Dr Padmavati, Director, SCARF for her support and kind foreword.

INTRODUCTION

This is part of a cognitive behaviour therapy book series programme. This book is for specifically tackling depression.

Designed specifically for the busy and hardworking who want to take control of their life and do something positive about it.

The slides will be easy to go through several times a day. You will be able to use the techniques as often as you want.

COGNITIVE BEHAVIOUR THERAPY

INVENTED BY PSYCHIATRIST BECK IN 1960

COGNITIVE BEHAVIOUR THERAPY (CBT) IS USED ALONG WITH MEDICATIONS WIDELY WORLD WIDE TO TREAT DEPRESSION

COGNITIVE PART OF THE THERAPY

TARGETS

NEGATIVE (SAD) THOUGHTS

AND THINKING ERRORS

BEHAVIOUR PART OF THE THERAPY

TARGETS

BEHAVIOURS THAT ARISE AS A RESULT OF THE NEGATIVE (SAD) THOUGHTS AND THINKING ERRORS

SAD THOUGHTS
(NEGATIVE AUTOMATIC THOUGHTS)

YOU GET MORE THAN 70,000 THOUGHTS PER DAY

SAD MOOD CAUSES SAD THOUGHTS AND VICE VERSA

SAD THOUGHTS CAN AFFECT THE WAY YOU BEHAVE

SAD THOUGHTS CAN AFFECT THE WAY YOU GET ALONG WITH PEOPLE

IDENTIFY YOUR SAD THOUGHTS

SAD THOUGHTS	HAPPY THOUGHTS
"I AM NOT GOOD ENOUGH"	"I AM GOOD AT WHAT I DO"
"I AM WORTHLESS"	"I AM VALUABLE"
"NOBODY LIKES ME"	"MANY PEOPLE LIKE ME"
"EVERYTHING IS MY FAULT"	"THERE ARE SEVERAL REASONS WHY EVENTS HAPPEN IN A CERTAIN WAY"
"I AM A FAILURE"	"I AM A SUCCESS IN MY LIFE"

IDENTIFY YOUR SAD THOUGHTS

SAD THOUGHTS	HAPPY THOUGHTS
"I WISH I WERE DEAD"	"LIFE IS INTERESTING"
"THINGS ARE GOING TO GET WORSE"	"I AM HOPEFUL OF MY FUTURE"
"LIFE HAS NO MEANING"	"LIFE IS FUN"
"SOMETHING IS WRONG WITH ME"	"I AM A HEALTHY PERSON"
"I FEEL TIRED ALL THE TIME"	"I AM FULL OF ENERGY"

MANAGE YOUR SAD THOUGHTS
YOU CAN _DEFUSE_ THE THOUGHTS

THANK THE MIND -
FOR EVERY SAD THOUGHT; KEEP SAYING
"THANK YOU, MIND"

WRITE DOWN YOUR SAD THOUGHTS AND SING IT ALOUD IN YOUR FAVOURITE NURSERY RHYME TUNE

THINK ABOUT ABSURD AND FUNNY OUTCOMES TO YOUR SAD THOUGHTS AND SEE THE LIGHT SIDED VIEW OF THE SITUATION

IMAGINE THAT YOUR SAD THOUGHTS ARE TAKING A WALK OUT OF YOUR MIND

JUMBLE UP THE WORDS OF YOUR SAD THOUGHTS TILL THEY SEEM ABSURD AND LOSE THEIR MEANING

THINK OF YOUR SAD THOUGHTS AS A NEWS TICKER THAT MOVES ALONG THE SCREEN UNDER THE NEWS

MANAGE YOUR SAD THOUGHTS
YOU CAN _ACCEPT_ THE THOUGHTS

DEVISE YOUR OWN "ACCEPTANCE MANTRA" AND ACCEPT YOUR SAD THOUGHTS WITHOUT ANY CONDITIONS

DESCRIBE YOUR SAD THOUGHTS AS YOU WOULD DESCRIBE A PHYSICAL OBJECT- THE SIZE, WEIGHT, VOLUME, COLOUR, TEXTURE AND SO FORTH

SIT WITH YOUR EYES CLOSED FOR A FEW MINUTES AND ACCEPT YOUR SAD THOUGHTS THAT COMES INTO YOUR MIND WITH ABSOLUTELY NO RESISTANCE

DO NOT INVEST EMOTIONS IN YOUR SAD THOUGHTS

ACCEPT YOUR THOUGHTS BUT DO NOT BE DEFEATED BY THEM

MANAGE YOUR SAD THOUGHTS

DISTRACT YOURSELF

DESTROY YOUR SAD THOUGHTS
WRITE THEM DOWN AND TEAR THE PAPER

DISPLAY POSITIVE SELF-TALK

MANAGE YOUR SAD THOUGHTS

TREAT YOURSELF TODAY

(Watch A Movie, Eat Out, Take A Long Bike Ride or Go to The Beach)

"Thank you" is the best prayer that one can say

NAME ONE THING YOU ARE GRATEFUL FOR TODAY

IMAGINE YOURSELF TO BE A LAWYER AND ARGUE AGAINST YOUR SAD THOUGHTS

Close your eyes and recount the last time you were happy.

Think about the thoughts you had.

What feelings and emotions did you experience?

MANAGE YOUR SAD THOUGHTS

ABCD METHOD
EXAMPLE - 1

A - ACTIVATING EVENT	Eg: A colleague Ignoring you
B - BELIEFS ABOUT THE EVENT	Eg: "I am an insignificant person"
C - CONSEQUENCES ABOUT THE EVENT	Eg: Losing confidence in yourself
D - DISPUTE THE EVENT	Eg: "He would not have seen me and did not ignore me deliberately"

MANAGE YOUR SAD THOUGHTS

ABCD METHOD
EXAMPLE - 2

A - ACTIVATING EVENT	Eg: Your girlfriend calls off the relationship
B - BELIEFS ABOUT THE EVENT	Eg: "I am not a lovable person"
C - CONSEQUENCES ABOUT THE EVENT	Eg: Feeling sad and angry
D - DISPUTE THE EVENT	Eg: "There are several reasons why the relationship did not work out. It's not because I am unlovable"

IDENTIFY AND CHALLENGE YOUR THINKING ERRORS

A lot of pain we are dealing with are actually only thoughts - Unknown

Thinking errors are faulty patterns of thinking that are **NOT** in keeping with actual facts

IDENTIFY AND CHALLENGE YOUR THINKING ERRORS

DO YOU THINK BLACK & WHITE?	**REMEMBER- THERE IS ALWAYS GREY**

For Example:

Do you think....

"If I don't get this job then I am a complete failure"

Make a mental note of the various times when you were successful in school, college, etc. You are not a failure just because you did not get this job.

IDENTIFY AND CHALLENGE YOUR THINKING ERRORS

DO YOU FILTER OUT THE HAPPY EVENTS AND FOCUS ONLY ON THE SAD ONES	RE-THINK - RE-FOCUS - RE-LIVE THE MOMENT HAPPILY

For Example:

Do you think....

"I am so upset by the sarcastic comment given by a guest about my dressing sense in the party"

Now rethink the whole event but with ONLY the happy moments and without the sad moments or comments.

Was the event mostly happy apart from the one comment?

IDENTIFY AND CHALLENGE YOUR THINKING ERRORS

DO YOU FORTUNE TELL? **DO YOU JUMP TO CONCLUSIONS?**	**LOOK AT THE FACTS VERSUS FICTION**
For Example: Do you think…. "I will _definitely_ fail in my exams"	Why do you think that? How have you prepared? What can you do to prepare well rather than focussing on the negative outcome?

IDENTIFY AND CHALLENGE YOUR THINKING ERRORS

DO YOU MIND READ?	NEVER ASSUME
For Example:	
"I _know_ that the manager thinks I am stupid"	Think about whether they have actually said anything to that effect?
"I _know_ that everyone thinks I am a loser"	What is the actual evidence that they think about you this way?

IDENTIFY AND CHALLENGE YOUR THINKING ERRORS

DO YOU OVERGENERALIZE A SIMPLE ISSUE?

THINK "IS THERE ANOTHER POINT OF VIEW?"

For Example:

Do you think...

"My husband was angry with me for cooking a bad meal. I know that he always hates me and doesn't like whatever I do"

Just because he did not like one meal, it does not mean he doesn't like other aspects about you.

Is there another point of view to this situation?

Is your inference too broad?

IDENTIFY AND CHALLENGE YOUR THINKING ERRORS

DO YOU GIVE YOURSELF LABELS?

AVOID LABELS

For Example:

Do you think…

"I divorced my husband; so, I am a _bad mom_"

Avoid labels like _bad mom._

Reflect whether you are really a bad mom and the reasons why you had to divorce.

Think whether the divorce has had a positive impact on your children.

IDENTIFY AND CHALLENGE YOUR THINKING ERRORS

DO YOU MAGNIFY OR MINIMIZE A SITUATION?	CHALLENGE THE THINKING
For Example: Do you think… "Since my spouse has died, I have nothing to look forward to in life"	How have others coped in similar situations? What are the other blessings in your life? Are there other aspects in life you can look forward to?

IDENTIFY AND CHALLENGE YOUR THINKING ERRORS

DO YOU PERSONALISE EVENTS?

THERE ARE ALWAYS OTHER POSSIBILITIES TO A SITUATION

For Example:

Do you think…

"My boyfriend went on holiday by himself without me. This is because he doesn't love me anymore"

Are you reading too much into this event?

Are there other explanations for him going on holiday by himself without you?

Is your thinking the most probable explanation?

IDENTIFY AND CHALLENGE YOUR THINKING ERRORS

IS YOUR THINKING CATASTROPHIC?

THERE ARE ALWAYS OTHER MILDER OUTCOMES

For Example:
Do you think....

"My back pain is so bad that I will end up in a wheel chair and I will not be able to work or pay my bills and will end up on the streets".

Is the situation really that bad?

What is the most likely outcome of your back pain?

Could there be any positive and milder outcomes to this situation?

SELF – HELP EXERCISES

1. DEDICATED WORRY TIMES

2. IMAGERY

3. NAME THE THOUGHT / NAME THE FEELING

4. MINDFULNESS

5. BREATHE MINDFULLY

6. PROGRESSIVE MUSCLE RELAXATION

7. PLEASANT ACTIVITIES

8. GROUNDING 5

EXERCISE - 1
DEDICATED WORRY TIMES

SET 10 MINUTES
MORNING AND EVENING

What to do during the dedicated worry times?

- Pick ONE worry
- ONLY worry for 10 minutes
- DO NOT distract, problem solve or think positively
- DO dwell on the negativity and feel anxious

EXERCISE - 2
IMAGERY

- Close your eyes for 5 minutes.
- Imagine that you are in your favourite holiday destination
- e.g., a beach, enjoying sunset, green parks

Describe what you can see

Describe what you can hear

Describe what you can feel

Describe what you can taste

EXERCISE - 3
NAME THE THOUGHT
NAME THE FEELING

Set an alarm on your phone every 3-4 hours.

Sit still for 5 minutes.

Notice your thoughts and emotions for 5 minutes

Name your emotions and thoughts

Eg: I _fear_ the sea; I feel _angry_ with my spouse

EXERCISE - 4
MINDFULNESS

MORNING: "BE PRESENT" WITH YOUR FIRST CUP OF TEA:
Notice the _taste_ of sweetness of your morning tea
Revel in the _smell_ and _colour_ of the tea.
Give a break to the "autopilot" and spend a full 10 minutes only enjoying your first cup of tea.

LUNCH: "BE PRESENT" IN THE PLACE:
Go to a different place for lunch
Sit by the window
Take in the view- be it a busy road, kids scurrying around or the serenity of the mountains.

EVENING: "BE PRESENT" WITH YOUR THOUGHTS:
Imagine that you are standing in a bus stop
Watch the buses stop and pass by without alighting any of those buses.
Use this analogy to watch your thoughts as a bystander without involving yourself emotionally.

EXERCISE - 5
BREATHE MINDFULLY

FIND A SPOT AND SIT ON A CUSHION

SCAN YOUR BODY AND FREE THE TENSION

INHALE AND EXHALE FOR A FEW MINUTES

NOTICE YOUR BREATH. DO NOT FORCE IT

EXERCISE - 6
PROGRESSIVE MUSCLE RELAXATION

Starting from your toes, tense each muscle group for 5-10 seconds and relax for double the time

FEEL a wave of relaxation as you release that tension

VISUALISE the relaxation

BREATHE normally throughout the exercise

EXERCISE - 7
PLEASANT ACTIVITES

Do an activity that make you feel good like.......

Watching the sunrise or sunset	Listening to music
Going to the movies	Helping someone
Going to the Temple	Praying
Cleaning the room	Walking
Talking to friends	Listening to jokes

EXERCISE - 8
THE GROUNDING 5

Name 5 things you can SEE right now

Name 4 things you can FEEL right now

Name 3 things you can HEAR right now

Name 2 things you can SMELL right now

Name 1 things you can TASTE right now

EXPAND YOUR SOCIAL CONNECTIONS

Start small and accept invitations to meet people.
Make people feel comfortable

Volunteer.
Do not judge people

Try to meet the friends of your friends

Be open minded and genuine.
Be yourself

Try to keep in touch with friends.
Help them if required

MANAGE YOUR EXPECTATIONS
Your expectations of others

For Example:

You place expectations on your child to be a topper in the state exam

Your expectations of others may set yourself up for disappointment and make your happiness and peace conditional on your child fulfilling those expectations

MANAGE YOUR EXPECTATIONS
Other's expectations of you

MAY MAKE YOU ANXIOUS

INADEQUATE

FRUSTRATED

MANAGE YOUR EXPECTATIONS

SET CLEAR BOUNDARIES

BE REALISTIC ABOUT WHAT YOU CAN DELIVER

BE HONEST AND SPECIFIC

IDENTIFY YOUR COMMUNICATION STYLE
PASSIVE STYLE OF COMMUNICATION

Are you unable to express what you feel because you feel others are superior to you?

Are you unable to express your opinion, rights and views openly?

Do you struggle with eye contact and have a slumped body posture?

Do you speak softly and allow people to interfere with your rights?

This style of communication can lead to frustration, resentment or low mood

IDENTIFY YOUR COMMUNICATION STYLE
AGGRESSIVE STYLE OF COMMUNICATION

Are you hostile, angry and think that you are superior to others?

Do you use a loud voice and intimidate others to get your point across?

Do you humiliate, criticize or dominate others?

Do you blame others instead of taking responsibility?

This style of communication may lead to hurting others and alienating people

IDENTIFY YOUR COMMUNICATION STYLE
ASSERTIVE STYLE OF COMMUNICATION

Are you able to say what you feel without feeling bad?

Do you feel comfortable expressing your feelings without the pressure that you may be disliked for expressing them?

Do you feel comfortable saying "No"?

Can you speak in a firm and deliberate voice?

This style of communication leads to better adjustment, good social relationships and better self esteem

COMMUNICATE EFFECTIVELY

Nobody can make you feel inferior without your consent - Eleanor Roosevelt

Agree to disagree

Practice saying "no" respectfully
Do not explain why or apologise

INSTRUCT FIRMLY

USE "I" STATEMENTS OFTEN.

For e.g: "I want you to finish your homework by 1 pm"

Rehearse phrases and keep repeating them like a broken record

CONCLUSION

Develop attributes to combat stresses of life

FORGIVE WHOLEHEARTEDLY

BE GRATEFUL

ACCEPT IMPERFECTIONS

APPRECIATE PEOPLE

PRACTICE COMPASSION

EMBRACE UNCERTAINTY

Identify what you want to achieve in this lifetime, your 5-year goals and 6-month goals.

BE SPECIFIC and REALISTIC.

Write them down.

CONCLUSION

What would you like your epitaph to read?
Plan to live so you will be proud of your life when you die.

Avoid alcohol and long-term use of sleeping tablets.

Using COGNITIVE BEHAVIOUR THERAPY with medications will be an effective strategy to combat depression.

DO NOT think you have failed if you need to take medications.

FLASHCARDS FOR POSITIVE AFFIRMATIONS

I AM LOVED

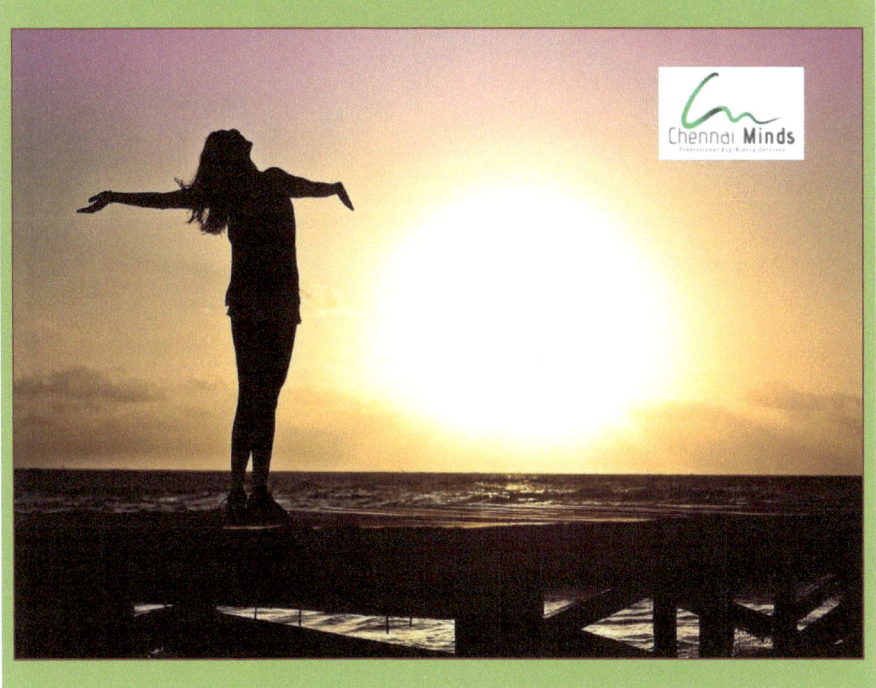

I AM HAPPY

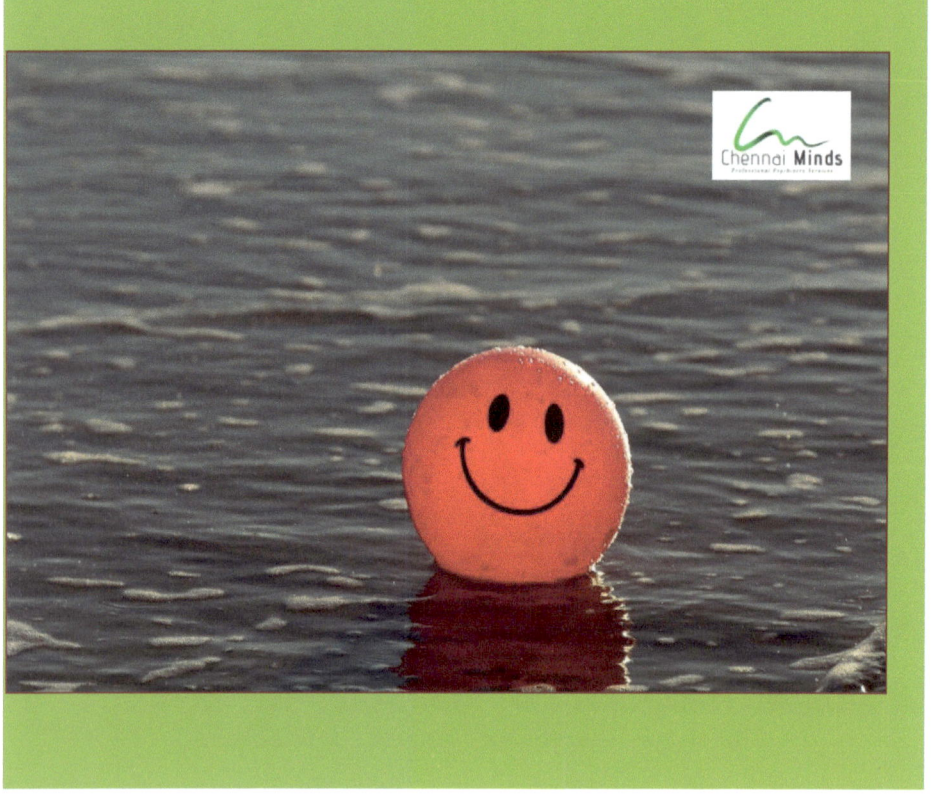

I AM ENTHUSIATIC

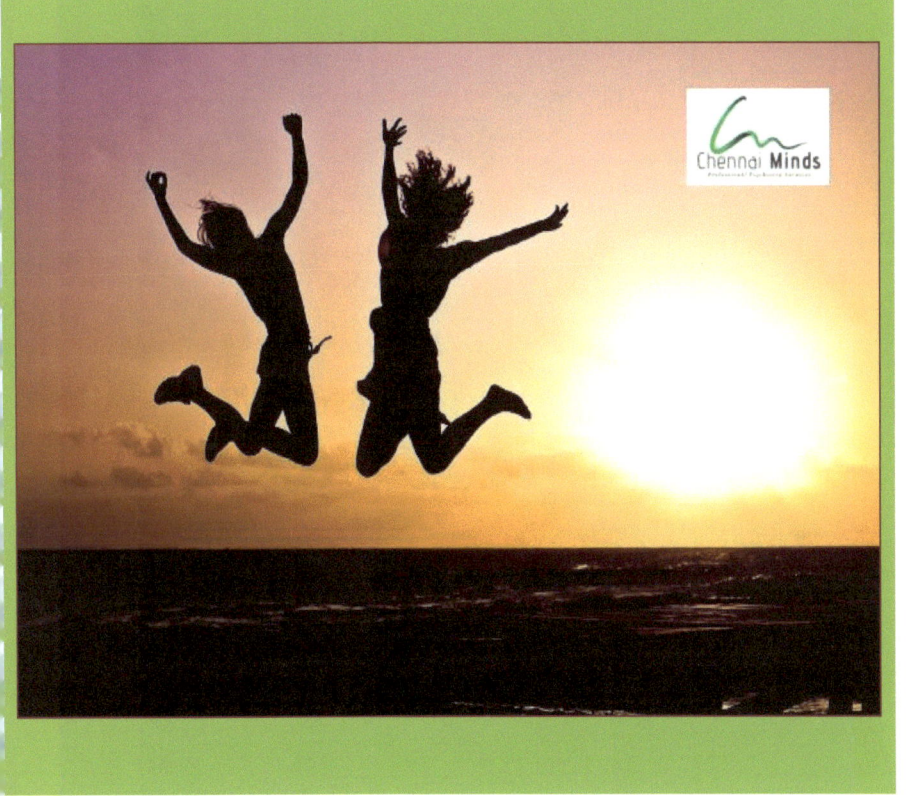

LIFE IS FUN

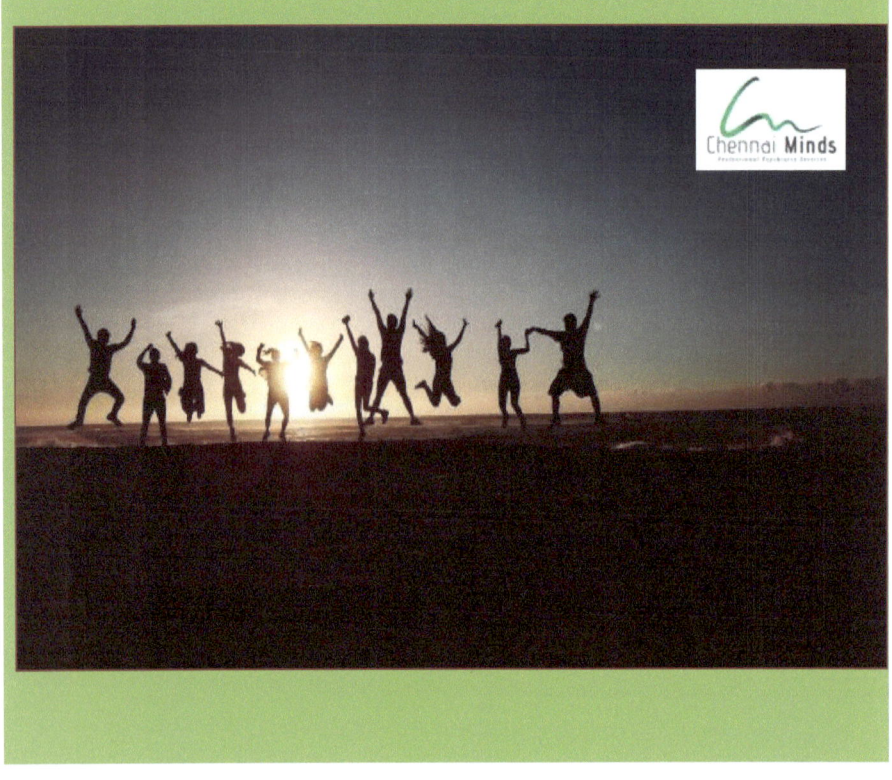

I AM FINE

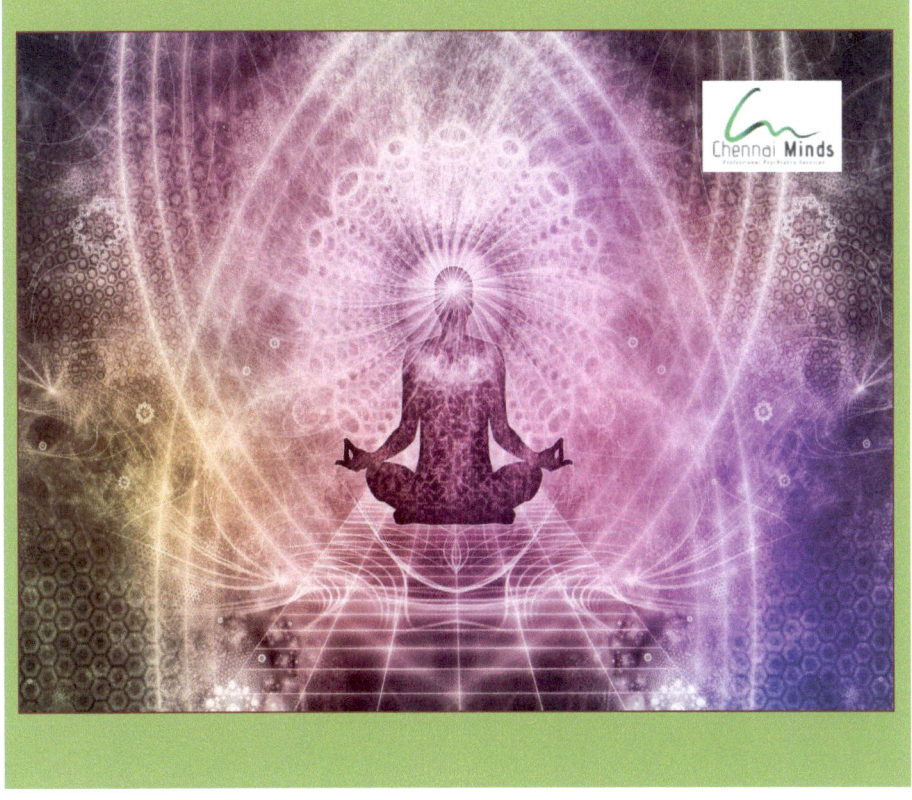

I AM GRATEFUL

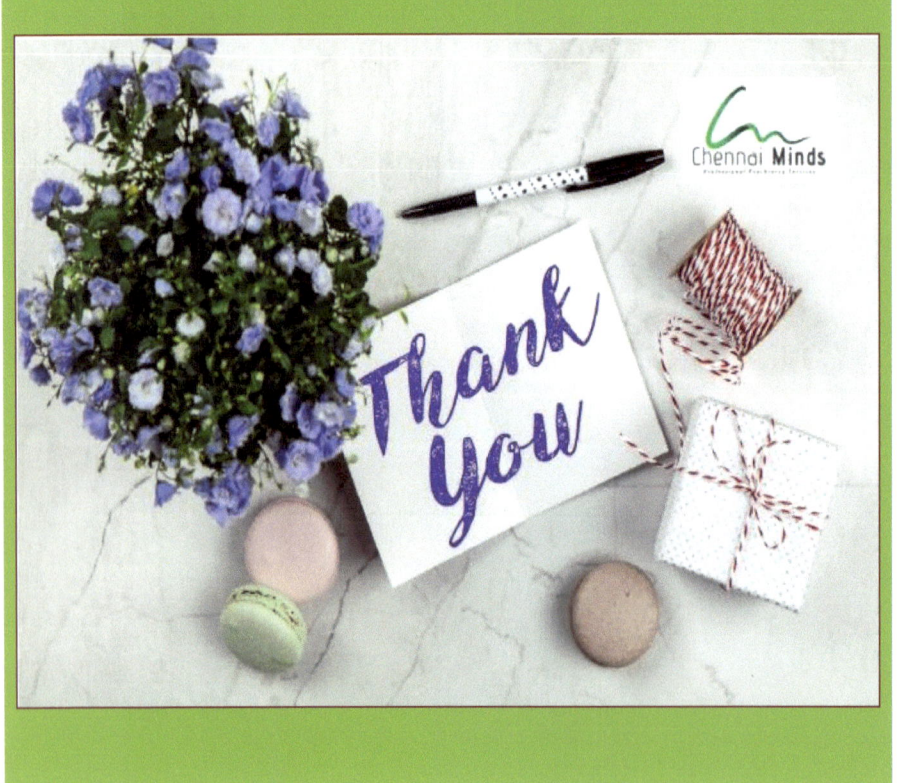

TODAY IS A SUCCESSFUL DAY

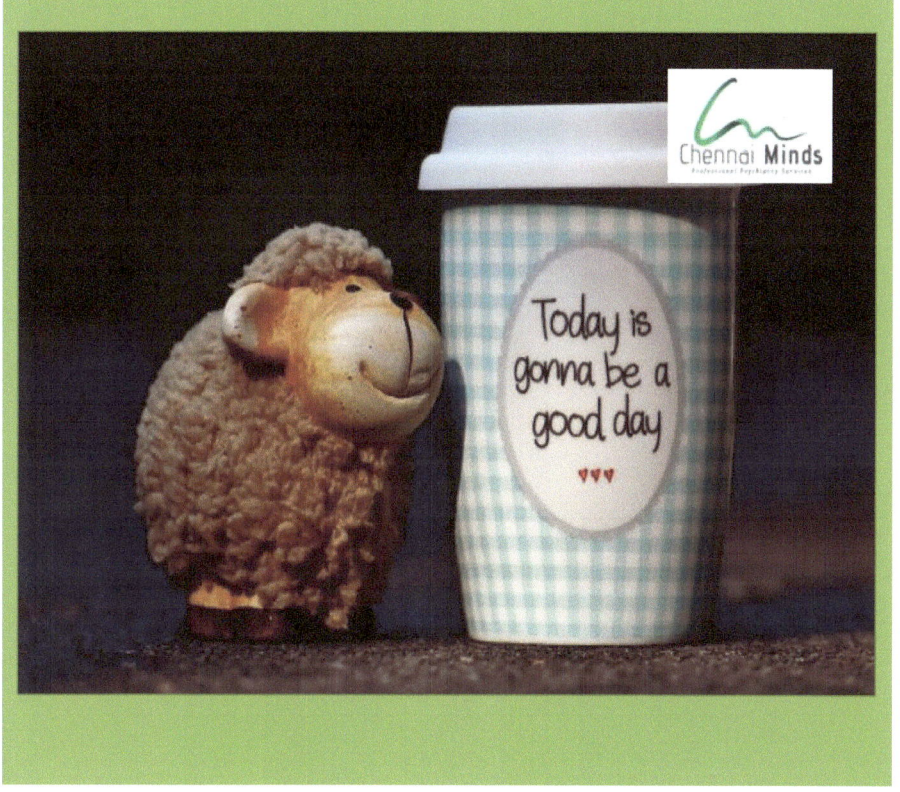

I AM VALUED

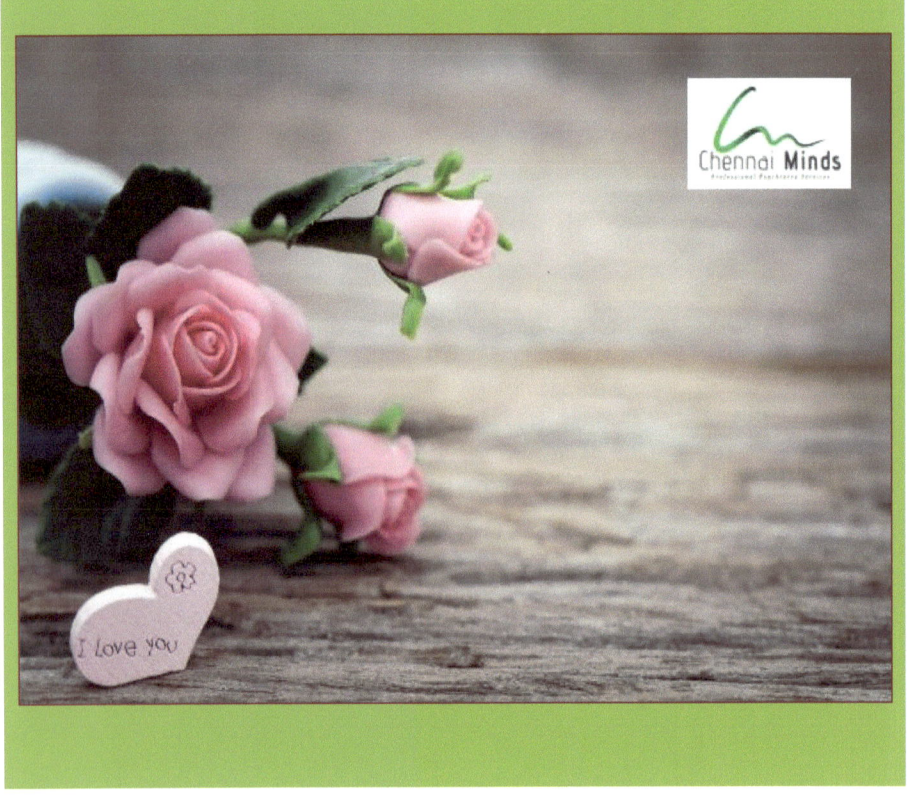

I AM STRONG

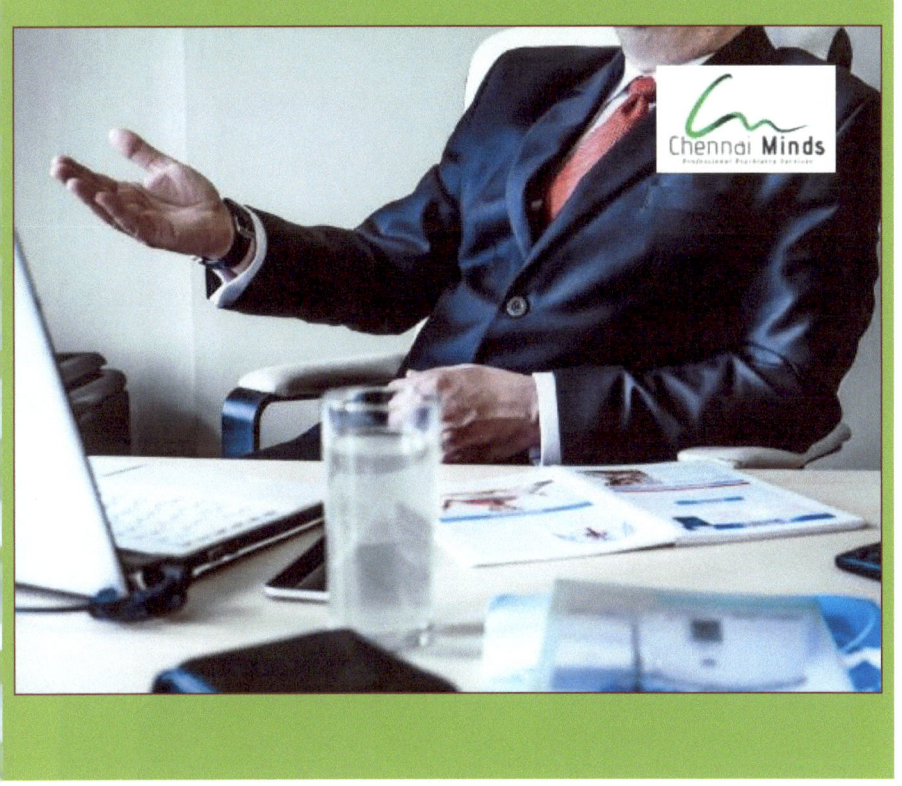

CONTACT US

WEBSITE: www.chennaiminds.com

EMAIL: drradhika@chennaiminds.com

WHATSAPP: +91 9677004220

FACEBOOK: http://www.facebook.com/chennaiminds

TWITTER: http://www.twitter.com/Chennai_Minds

LINKEDIN: http://www.linkedin.com/company/chennai-minds-official/

INSTAGRAM: http://www.instagram.com/Chennai_minds

YOUTUBE:
https://www.youtube.com/channel/UCrm6Rg6pYdI04pF7Q4R27ww

About Dr. Radhika ...

An alumnus of the prestigious Madras Medical College, Dr Radhika graduated MBBS from MMC, Chennai in the year 1999. Passionate about the holistic approach of treatment in psychiatry, she moved to the United Kingdom to pursue higher training in psychiatry. After receiving the MRCPsych (postgraduate degree in psychiatry) and CCT (super specialty qualifications in psychiatry) from UK, Dr. Radhika also received a higher research degree from UCL London (MSc in Psychiatric research).

Being born and bred in Chennai, Chennai has always been Dr. Radhika's final dream and destination. She was acutely aware of the shortage of psychiatry services in Chennai and decided to move back to her own birthplace with ambitions of bringing international standards of psychiatric care to the heart of Chennai.

She started CHENNAI MINDS (the initials CM to denote her beloved late father Mr. C. Murugesan). He was affectionately known as CM. Her father has been her role model and inspiration not only as a dedicated civil engineer but also as a human being with values and virtues worthy of emulation.

This book, Cognitive Behaviour Therapy for Depression, which is part of a series of self-help books, was born because Dr. Radhika was aware that patients did not find the time or resources to engage in therapy of 12 weeks and most self-help books were not simple or user friendly. Though this is not a substitute for therapy, these books will be a good start if you are struggling to bring yourself to a psychiatrist or in conjunction with psychiatric medications.

Other books in this series will soon be available including Cognitive Behavior therapy for obsessive compulsive disorder, Illness anxiety disorder, social anxiety disorder, panic disorder, Generalized Anxiety Disorder, alcohol dependence, etc. These books will be available in Tamil too.

Please send your queries and feedback to drradhika@chennaiminds.com

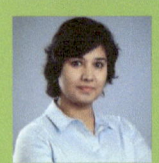

www.ingramcontent.com/pod-product-compliance
Lightning Source LLC
Chambersburg PA
CBHW040238220526
45473CB00001B/293